Strength Training For Beginners

Get Started Today

~ By My Girl Fit

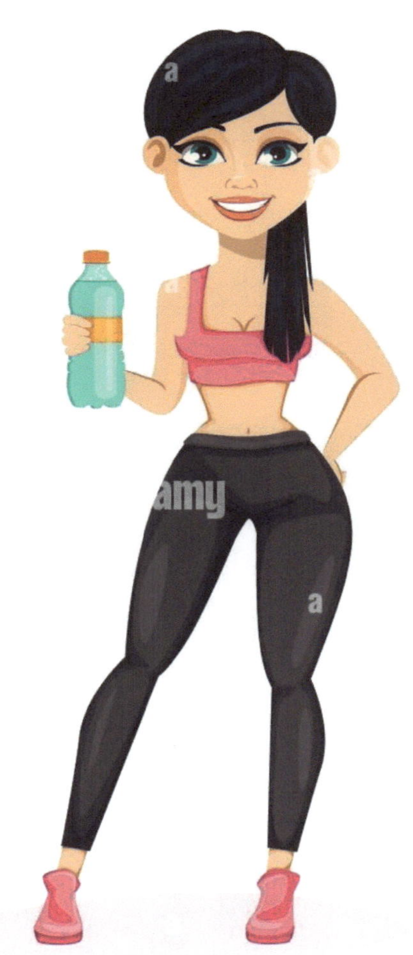

Table of Contents

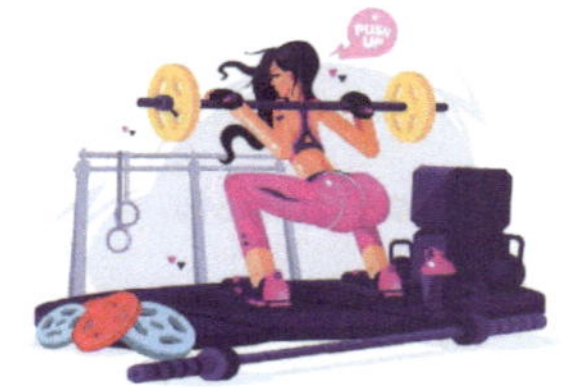

Welcome to the world of strength training! Strength training is a powerful way to improve your overall fitness and well-being, and it's an essential component of any fitness routine. Whether you're a seasoned athlete or just starting out, strength training can help you achieve your fitness goals and enjoy the many benefits that come with it.

In this ebook, we'll look at the different types of strength training, including free weights, cable machines, and yoga. We'll also provide guidance on proper form and technique, which are essential for getting the most out of your workouts and avoiding injury. Additionally, we'll provide tips for incorporating strength training into your busy schedule and making it a sustainable part of your fitness routine.

We'll cover all the aspects of strength training with free weights, cable machines, and yoga. We'll also provide guidance on proper nutrition and rest, which are essential for muscle growth and recovery.

Strength training can help you build muscle mass, increase your strength and flexibility, and enhance your athletic performance. Additionally, strength training can help you manage your weight, improve your bone density, and reduce your risk of injury.

Despite its many benefits, strength training is often misunderstood. Many people believe that strength training is only for bodybuilders or athletes, but the truth is that anyone can benefit from strength training. Whether you're a busy professional or a stay-at-home parent, strength training can help you improve your overall health and fitness and enhance your quality of life.

After reading this ebook through to the conclusion, you'll have a comprehensive understanding of strength training and how it can help you achieve your fitness goals. You'll also have the knowledge and tools you need to start your strength training journey and enjoy the many benefits that come with it.

So let's get started! In the first chapter, we'll explore the benefits of strength training with free weights.

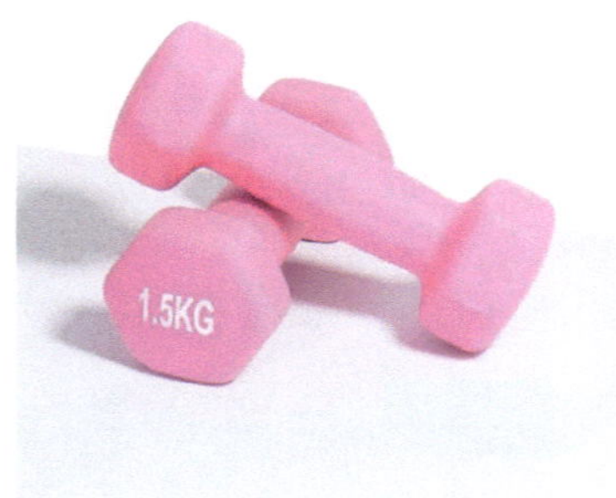

Free weights are a great way to build strength and muscle mass. They allow for a full range of motion and work multiple muscle groups at once. Here are some benefits of strength training with free weights:

- Increased muscle mass and strength

- Improved bone density

- Enhanced athletic performance

- Improved overall health and well-being

Some effective free weight exercises include:

- Squats

- Deadlifts

- Bench Press

- Rows

- Lunges

- Bicep Curls

- Tricep Extensions

Strength training with free weights is a great way to improve overall fitness. Free weights include dumbbells, barbells, and kettlebells, and they allow for a full range of motion and work multiple muscle groups at once.

Benefits of strength training with free weights include increased muscle mass and strength, improved bone density, enhanced athletic performance, and improved overall health and well-being.

Types of free weights include:

- Dumbbells: These are short bars with weights on each end and are great for exercises like bicep curls and tricep extensions.
- Barbells: These are longer bars with weights on each end and are great for exercises like squats and deadlifts.
- Kettlebells: These are weighted balls with a handle and are great for exercises like swings and cleans.

Exercises for each major muscle group include:

- Chest: bench press, dumbbell press, incline press

- Back: rows, lat pulldowns, deadlifts

- Shoulders: shoulder press, lateral raises, front raises

- Legs: squats, lunges, leg press

- Arms: bicep curls, tricep extensions, hammer curls

- Core: planks, Russian twists, leg raises

Tips for proper form and technique include:

- Start with light weights and gradually increase the weight as you become stronger.

- Use a full range of motion and avoid jerky movements.

- Keep your core engaged and your back straight.

- Breathe naturally and avoid holding your breath.

Sample workout routine:

Monday (Chest and Triceps):

- Barbell bench press (3 sets of 8-12 reps)

- Incline dumbbell press (3 sets of 10-15 reps)

- Tricep pushdowns (3 sets of 12-15 reps)

- Tricep dips (3 sets of 12-15 reps)

Wednesday (Back and Biceps):

- Pull-ups (3 sets of 8-12 reps)

- Barbell rows (3 sets of 8-12 reps)

- Dumbbell bicep curls (3 sets of 10-15 reps)

- Hammer curls (3 sets of 10-15 reps)

Friday (Legs and Shoulders):

- Squats (3 sets of 8-12 reps)

- Leg press (3 sets of 10-15 reps)

- Standing military press (3 sets of 8-12 reps)

- Lateral raises (3 sets of 10-15 reps)

In summary, strength training with free weights is a powerful way to improve overall fitness and well-being. It offers numerous benefits, including increased muscle mass and strength, improved bone density, enhanced athletic performance, and improved overall health and well-being. By incorporating free weight exercises into your fitness routine, you can improve your overall health and fitness, increase your strength and flexibility, and enhance your athletic performance.

Remember to always start with light weights and gradually increase the weight as you become stronger. It's also important to focus on proper form and technique, and to listen to your body and take rest days as needed. With consistency and dedication, you can achieve your fitness goals and enjoy the many benefits that come with strength training with free weights.

In the next chapter, we'll explore the benefits of strength training with cable machines. Cable machines offer a unique set of benefits and can be a great addition to your fitness routine.

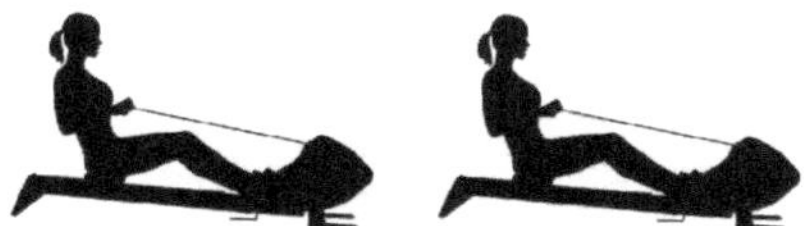

Strength training with cable machines is another effective way to build strength and target specific muscle groups. Cable machines provide a smooth and consistent resistance throughout the entire range of motion.

Benefits of strength training with cable machines include targeted muscle growth and strength, improved muscle tone and definition, enhanced athletic performance, and low-impact and easy on the joints.

Types of cable machines include:

- Chest press machine

- Shoulder press machine

- Lat pulldown machine

- Leg curl machine

Exercises for each major muscle group include:

- Chest: chest press, cable flyes

- Back: lat pulldowns, seated rows

- Shoulders: shoulder press, lateral raises

- Legs: leg curls, leg extensions

- Arms: bicep curls, tricep extensions

- Core: planks, Russian twists

Tips for proper form and technique include:

- Start with light weights and gradually increase the weight as you become stronger.

- Use a full range of motion and avoid jerky movements.

- Keep your core engaged and your back straight.

- Breathe naturally and avoid holding your breath.

Sample workout routine:

Monday (Chest and Triceps):

- Cable chest press (3 sets of 8-12 reps)

- Cable flyes (3 sets of 10-15 reps)

- Tricep pushdowns (3 sets of 12-15 reps)

- Tricep dips (3 sets of 12-15 reps)

Wednesday (Back and Biceps):

- Lat pulldowns (3 sets of 8-12 reps)

- Seated rows (3 sets of 10-15 reps)

- Bicep curls (3 sets of 10-15 reps)

- Hammer curls (3 sets of 10-15 reps)

Friday (Legs and Shoulders):

- Leg curls (3 sets of 8-12 reps)

- Leg extensions (3 sets of 10-15 reps)

- Shoulder press (3 sets of 8-12 reps)

- Lateral raises (3 sets of 10-15 reps)

Strength training with cable machines is a versatile and effective way to improve overall fitness and well-being. Cable machines offer a range of benefits, including increased muscle strength and endurance, improved muscle tone and definition, and enhanced athletic performance. By incorporating cable machine exercises into your fitness routine, you can improve your overall health and fitness, increase your strength and flexibility, and enhance your athletic performance.

Remember to always start with light weights and gradually increase the weight as you become stronger. It's also important to focus on proper form and technique, and to listen to your body and take rest days as needed. With consistency and dedication, you can achieve your fitness goals and enjoy the many benefits that come with strength training with cable machines.

In the following chapter, we'll explore the benefits of yoga for strength and flexibility. Yoga offers a unique set of benefits that can complement your strength training routine and improve your overall fitness and well-being. Let's take a look!

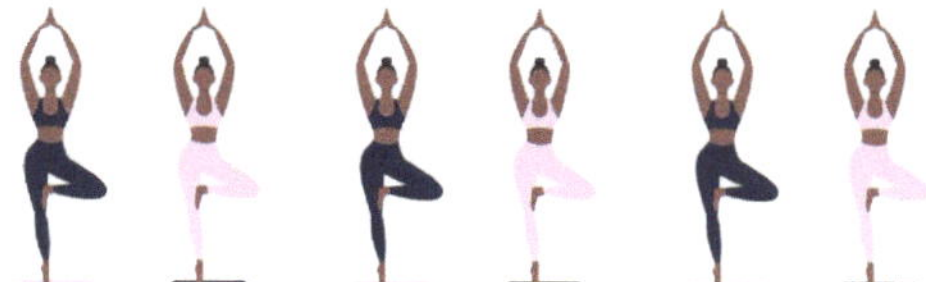

Yoga is a great way to improve flexibility, balance, and strength. It also provides many mental and emotional benefits, such as reduced stress and improved focus. Here are some benefits of yoga for strength and flexibility:

- Improved flexibility and range of motion

- Increased strength and muscle tone

- Enhanced balance and coordination

- Reduced stress and improved overall well-being

Some effective yoga poses for strength and flexibility include:

- Downward-Facing Dog

- Warrior II

- Triangle Pose

- Tree Pose

- Seated Forward Fold

- Plank Pose

Yoga is a holistic practice that combines physical postures, breathing techniques, and meditation to promote physical, mental, and emotional well-being. While often associated with flexibility and relaxation, yoga can also be a powerful tool for building strength and improving overall fitness.

Benefits of Yoga for Strength and Flexibility:

- Increased strength and flexibility

- Improved balance and coordination

- Enhanced muscle tone and definition

- Reduced muscle soreness and injury

- Improved overall physical fitness

Types of Yoga:

- Hatha Yoga: focuses on physical postures and breathing techniques

- Vinyasa Yoga: focuses on flowing movements and breathing techniques

- Ashtanga Yoga: focuses on fast-paced flowing movements and breathing techniques

- Restorative Yoga: focuses on relaxation and rejuvenation

Yoga Poses for Strength and Flexibility:

- Downward-Facing Dog: stretches hamstrings, calves, and spine

- Warrior II: strengthens legs and hips

- Triangle Pose: stretches hips, thighs, and spine

- Tree Pose: improves balance and focus

- Seated Forward Fold: stretches hamstrings, calves, and spine

- Plank Pose: strengthens arms, shoulders, and core

Tips for Starting a Yoga Practice:

- Start slow and gentle

- Listen to your body and modify or rest when needed

- Practice regularly for maximum benefits

- Focus on breathing and relaxation techniques

- Use props such as blocks, straps, and blankets for support

Sample Yoga Routine:

Monday (Beginner's Yoga):

- Downward-Facing Dog (5 breaths)

- Warrior II (5 breaths per side)

- Triangle Pose (5 breaths per side)

- Tree Pose (5 breaths per side)

- Seated Forward Fold (5 breaths)

- Plank Pose (5 breaths)

Wednesday (Intermediate Yoga):

- Sun Salutations (10 rounds)

- Warrior I (5 breaths per side)

- Triangle Pose (5 breaths per side)

- Side Plank Pose (5 breaths per side)

- Seated Forward Fold (5 breaths)

- Savasana (5 breaths)

Friday (Restorative Yoga):

- Legs Up The Wall Pose (10 breaths)

- Reclined Pigeon Pose (10 breaths per side)

- Reclined Spinal Twist Pose (10 breaths per side)

- Savasana (10 breaths)

Yoga is a powerful tool for building strength and improving flexibility. By incorporating yoga into your fitness routine, you can improve your overall physical fitness, increase your strength and flexibility, and reduce your risk of injury. Remember to start slow and gentle, listen to your body, and practice regularly for maximum benefits. With consistency and dedication, you can achieve your fitness goals and enjoy the many benefits that come with yoga.

In perhaps one of the most critical chapters of this ebook, we'll explore the importance of proper nutrition for strength training and overall fitness. Nutrition plays a vital role in muscle growth and recovery, and it's essential to fuel your body with the right foods to support your fitness goals.

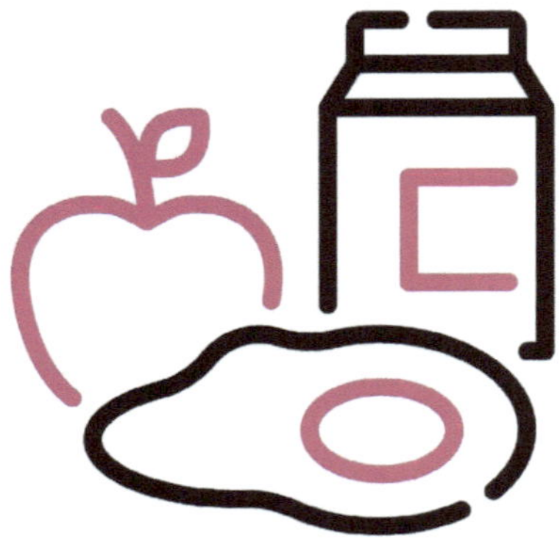

Proper nutrition is essential for strength training and muscle growth. A well-balanced diet provides the necessary building blocks for muscle recovery and growth. Nutrition, alone, leads to 80 percent of your total body composition. Important factors of a balanced diet included managing your nutrient sources.

Macronutrients:

- Protein: essential for muscle growth and repair

- Carbohydrates: provide energy for workouts

- Fat: provides energy and supports hormone production

Micronutrients:

- Vitamins: support muscle growth and recovery

- Minerals: support muscle function and recovery

Supplementation:

- Protein powder: convenient way to increase protein intake

- Creatine: increases strength and endurance

- Branched-Chain Amino Acids (BCAAs): reduces muscle soreness

Here are some nutrition tips and a sample meal plan to support your strength training goals:

- Eat enough protein to support muscle growth and repair

- Include complex carbohydrates in your diet for energy and recovery

- Healthy fats are essential for hormone production and overall health

- Stay hydrated by drinking plenty of water throughout the day

Some effective nutrition strategies include:

- Meal planning and prep

- Post-workout nutrition

- Supplementation (protein powder, creatine, etc.)

Sample meal plan:

Breakfast:

- 3 whole eggs

- 2 egg whites

- 2 slices whole wheat toast

- 1 cup oatmeal

Snack:

- 1 scoop protein powder

- 1 cup Greek yogurt

- 1 cup mixed berries

Lunch:

- 4 oz grilled chicken breast

- 1 cup brown rice

- 1 cup steamed vegetables

Snack:

- 1 medium apple

- 2 tbsp almond butter

Dinner:

- 6 oz grilled salmon

- 1 cup sweet potato

- 1 cup steamed broccoli

Post-workout nutrition:

- Consume protein and carbohydrates within 30 minutes of workout

- Include a source of protein and carbohydrates in post-workout meal

Proper nutrition is essential for strength training and overall fitness. By fueling your body with the right foods, you can support muscle growth and recovery, improve your performance, and achieve your fitness goals. Remember to focus on whole, unprocessed foods, stay hydrated, and avoid sugary and processed foods. With a balanced diet and a consistent training routine, you can achieve optimal fitness and overall well-being.

Next up, we'll cover the importance of rest and recovery for strength training and overall fitness. Rest and recovery are critical components of the fitness equation, and it's essential to prioritize them to avoid injury and achieve optimal results.

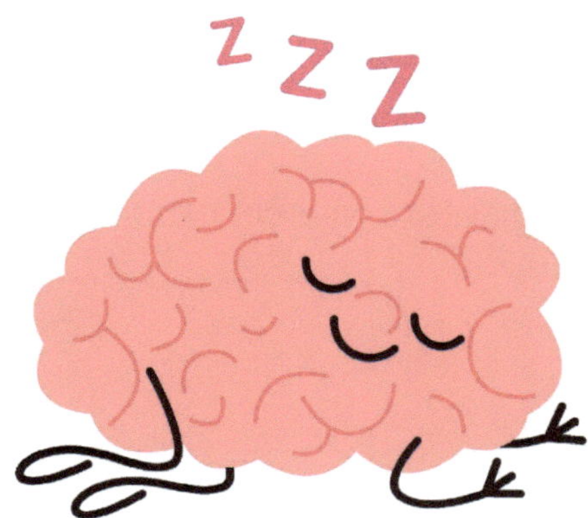

Rest and recovery are critical components of the fitness equation. While exercise is essential for building strength and improving fitness, rest and recovery are equally important for allowing your body to repair and adapt to the demands of exercise.

Benefits of Rest and Recovery:

- Allows muscles to repair and rebuild

- Reduces muscle soreness and fatigue

- Improves performance and reduces risk of injury

- Enhances overall physical and mental well-being

Types of Rest and Recovery:

- Passive rest: complete cessation of exercise

- Active rest: low-intensity exercise such as yoga or walking

- Cross-training: alternative exercises that target different muscle groups

Tips for Rest and Recovery:

- Listen to your body and take rest days as needed

- Prioritize sleep and aim for 7-9 hours per night

- Use foam rolling and self-myofascial release to reduce muscle tension

- Incorporate stretching and yoga to improve flexibility and reduce muscle soreness

Sample Rest and Recovery Routine:

Monday (Rest day):

- No exercise

- Focus on stretching and foam rolling

Tuesday (Active rest):

- Yoga or walking

- Low-intensity exercise to promote blood flow and recovery

Wednesday (Cross-training):

- Alternative exercise such as swimming or cycling

- Targets different muscle groups to allow for recovery

Thursday (Rest day):

- No exercise

- Focus on stretching and foam rolling

Friday (Active rest):

- Yoga or walking

- Low-intensity exercise to promote blood flow and recovery

Rest and recovery are crucial components of a well-rounded fitness routine. By prioritizing rest and recovery, you can improve your performance, reduce your risk of injury, and enhance your overall physical and mental well-being. Remember to listen to your body, prioritize sleep, and incorporate stretching and foam rolling into your routine. With a balanced approach to exercise and recovery, you can achieve optimal fitness and overall health.

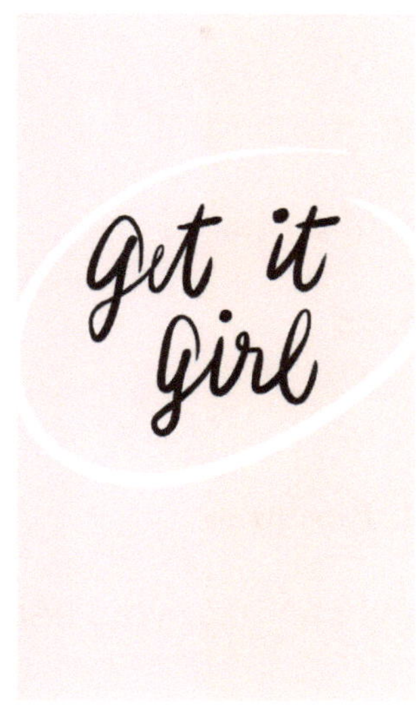

In conclusion, strength training with free weights, cable machines, and yoga, combined with proper nutrition and rest, is a powerful way to achieve overall fitness and well-being. It's important to remember that consistency and dedication are key, and to always consult with a healthcare professional before starting any new exercise program. Always listen to your body before, during and after a workout.

By incorporating strength training into your fitness routine, you can improve your overall health and fitness, increase your strength and flexibility, and enhance your athletic performance. Additionally, strength training can help you manage your weight, improve your bone density, and reduce your risk of injury.

Remember to always start slow and gradually increase the intensity and difficulty of your workouts as you become stronger. It's also important to listen to your body and take rest days as needed, as proper rest and recovery are essential for muscle growth and repair.

In addition to strength training, proper nutrition is essential for muscle growth and recovery. Make sure to consume a balanced diet that includes plenty of protein, carbohydrates, and healthy fats, and avoid sugary and processed foods.

Finally, remember to stay hydrated and get enough sleep each night. Adequate hydration and sleep are essential for muscle recovery and growth, and can help you feel your best.

By following these tips and incorporating strength training into your fitness routine, you can achieve your fitness goals and enjoy the many benefits that come with it. Remember to always consult with a healthcare professional before starting any new exercise program, and to listen to your body and take rest days as needed.

In addition to the physical benefits of strength training, it can also have a profound impact on your mental and emotional health. Lifting weights and doing yoga can help reduce stress and anxiety, improve your mood, and enhance your overall sense of well-being.

Remember, strength training is a journey, and it's important to be patient and consistent. Don't get discouraged if you don't see results right away – keep pushing forward, and you will eventually start to see the benefits of your hard work.

In conclusion, strength training with free weights, cable machines, and yoga, combined with proper nutrition and rest, is a powerful way to achieve overall fitness and well-being. Remember to always consult with a healthcare professional before starting any new exercise program, and to listen to your body and take rest days as needed. With consistency and dedication, you can achieve your fitness goals and enjoy the many benefits that come with it.